CBD Oil for Pain Relief: 2 Manuscripts - How to Naturally Remedy Physical Pain & Anxiety

By Lauren Marshall

This books contains 2 Manuscripts:

Hemp Oil and CBD: Your Guide to Using Natural Oils for Physical Injuries, Mental Health & General Wellbeing

Essential Oils: Discover the Drug-Free, Safe & Inexpensive Way to Combat Anxiety & Stress with 20 DIY Recipes

Medical Disclaimer

This book is not intended as a substitute for the medical advice of physicians. The reader should regularly consult a physician in matters relating to his/her health and particularly with respect to any symptoms that may require diagnosis or medical attention. Any recommendations given in this book are not a substitute for medical advice.

Contents

Hemp Oil and CBD

Your Guide to Using Natural Oils for Physical Injuries, Mental Health & General Wellbeing

By Lauren Marshall

Introduction: Big Pharma vs Natural Healing

The $450 billion a year pharmaceutical industry is responsible for the creation, distribution and marketing of what is commonly thought of as medicine. Everything from the Aspirin we take to relieve a headache to the Tylenol used to lower a fever qualifies as medicine. Likewise, life-saving drugs such as insulin, epinephrine, Digitalis, as well as penicillin and other vaccines for deadly illnesses fall underneath the blanket term "Big Pharma."

While there are a large number of "Big Pharma" companies in North America, the top three are Johnson and Johnson, Pfizer and Merck and Company.
There are a number of big pharmaceutical companies in America, with the top three being Johnson & Johnson (which did over eighteen billion in sales during the last quarter of 2016), Pfizer (averaged around thirteen billion) and Merck & Company (averaged a relatively minor ten billion in sales).

These three companies are not only incredibly profitable, they are also immensely powerful. They literally hold people's lives and health in their hands, as they control the rights to the medication that these same people need to function from day to day or even to survive. A diabetic must have access to insulin in order to regulate their blood sugar, just as a patient with severe depression may rely upon medication to stabilize their mood swings and control their anxiety. The pharmaceutical companies which manufacture and distribute these medications are able to put a price tag on the health and well-being of other humans. If a person is in need of a certain medication but cannot afford it, the pharmaceutical company does not drop their prices to accommodate the patient's needs. Rather, the patient must find a way to come up with the money needed, or they simply have to go without, often at the detriment of their physical or mental health.

It goes without saying that Big Pharma is an incredibly profitable industry for the key players involved. While the top three pharmaceutical companies did over three trillion dollars' worth of business in 2016 with a profit margin of over twenty percent, it is estimated that seven out of ten drugs released by these companies are too expensive to be realistic for the general population. With the giant profit margins these companies experience, they are facing intense backlash from the average citizen who urges them to drop their prices in order to allow easier access to necessary, life-saving drugs.

So how do they get away with it? Plain and simple, they use the free market and the concept of supply and demand. For example, say a Big Pharma company develops a drug that they know will help save multiple lives and/or improve overall physical health. This product will understandably be in very high demand. The more in demand a product is, the more a company can charge to the consumer. What this unfortunately boils down to, is that the patients who are most in need of a particular medication, such as chemotherapy for cancer treatment, almost always ends up paying far more for their drugs than it actually costs the pharmaceutical company to manufacture and market them.

Not only do Big Pharma companies regularly engage in price gouging and profiteering, there are also serious doubts as to whether or not these pharmaceutical companies are actually working to help improve the health of the citizens they claim to serve. Many companies have been accused of tampering with clinical drug trial results, meaning that they are seeking to emphasize the positive aspects of a certain medication while blatantly glossing over many potentially serious or even fatal side effects that that same drug may carry.

Big Pharma is also responsible for the manufacture and marketing of opioids and other powerful painkillers. Not long ago, these drugs were given freely to patients to treat the physical discomfort associated with recovering from surgery, broken bones, chronic pain issues, etc. While these drugs were certainly effective at relieving pain, they also came with a heavy risk of patient dependency and addiction. The pharmaceutical companies that created these drugs and pushed them upon the general population did not make physicians or patients fully aware of the extreme potential for addiction and resulting health issues. Not surprisingly, this has led to a huge epidemic of opioid addiction in the United States. In fact, opioid addiction numbers have risen a staggering 500% over the past 5 years. This contributes to more than 50,000 deaths per yar among US adults. Many patients who became inadvertently dependent upon prescription drugs following some sort of serious illness or medical crisis, were never properly warned about the potential for developing a chemical dependence upon the drug.

However, recent decades have found many Americans turning away from traditional medicine in an attempt to seek out more natural remedies of maintaining and improving the health. It is not just the fact that Big Pharma so blatantly takes advantage of the same population they claim to serve. Many prescription drugs carry potentially serious side effects or interactions with them that are not experienced with more natural methods of healing.

Many forms of alternative healing, such as aromatherapy, reiki, hypnosis and herbology are finally beginning to make their way into mainstream consciousness rather than being relegated strictly to the realm of new-age hippies. Individuals are finally able to freely access information in order to educate themselves about the various options they have available to them rather than believing they must simply content themselves with following the doctor's orders.

Far and away, one of the most talked about developments in natural healing has been the increased interest in medical marijuana as well as Hemp oil and Cannabidiol, more commonly referred to as CBD. While marijuana, hemp and CBD are all products of the same Cannabis plant, they have very different properties which will be discussed in depth later on in this book. For now, suffice to say that even though Hemp Oil & CBD is far different than marijuana, Big Pharma is very invested in keeping all forms of hemp use illegal, as it profits them greatly to do so.

Pharmaceutical companies are vehemently opposed to legalizing medical marijuana as well conducting research into the effectiveness of CBD hemp oil. This opposition is in the face of a tremendous amount of evidence which shows the beneficial effects that both marijuana and CBD oil possess. Marijuana, for example, has been proven to dramatically improve patient health in instances of Post-Traumatic Stress Disorder, Obsessive Compulsive Disorder as well as with clinical depression. Medical marijuana is a powerful anti-emetic, meaning that it can greatly benefit those with chronic nausea, being particularly effective for patients suffering from the unpleasant side-effects of chemotherapy. Marijuana is also able to stimulate the appetite, which helps patients recovering from anorexia, bulimia or other eating disorders.

CBD hemp oil is being touted by many users as the new "miracle drug" due to its many powerful healing qualities. CBD oil not only helps alleviate seizures, tremors and overall nerve and body pain, it can also calm feelings of anxiety, lessen the symptoms of ADD/ADHD and has even been shown in some studies to decrease or even eliminate the growth of cancer cells and tumors.

This begs the obvious question - if cannabis is so great, then why isn't it legal everywhere? Why don't we have free reign to cultivate, purchase and sell cannabis just as we would any other staple, such as cotton, wheat or soy?

The pure, simply reason as to why Big Pharma fights so mightily against the medical marijuana and hemp industry is not out of concern for the citizens it claims to help. In fact, it is the exact opposite. Big Pharma's resistance towards cannabis is motivated by nothing more than pure, simple monetary motivations. Hemp is relatively easy to grow, meaning that if it were legal, just about anyone in the United States would be able to have unlimited access to the plant. These pharmaceutical companies are very well aware that many patients would turn away from their reliance upon prescription drugs if another viable, legal alternative was made available to them. Thus, Big Pharma continues to block public access to hemp and marijuana out of concern in protecting their own interests. As long as cannabis remains illegal, doctors are forced to stick to prescribing the drugs that the pharmaceutical companies let the prescribe, and Big Pharma keeps on making a ridiculous amount of money off sick Americans each year.

Chapter One: Getting to Know Hemp

Hemp is a variety of Cannabis plant. It is grown strictly for its industrial use, as its fibers have been used to create functional, strong fibers for over ten thousand years. There is a wide variety of things that commercial hemp can be used for, including paper, clothing, rope, sails, textiles, etc.

Hemp has a long, contradictory history in the United States. Beginning in the 1700's, hemp was considered the number one most profitable crop in America. Colonists in Connecticut, Virginia and Massachusetts were required by law to grow hemp on their land, and faced heavy fines and even imprisonment if they neglected to do so. The hemp plant was so valuable during America's colonial days that it could even be exchanged much like money for goods and services.

The cultivation and sale of hemp was completely unregulated until the early 1900's. In 1914, the Harrison Act defined the use of marijuana, and therefore hemp, as a crime. In the next thirteen years, California, Louisiana, New York, Texas and Utah all outlawed marijuana as well. The increasing illegality of cannabis coupled with the invention of the cotton gin in the 1920's caused cotton to quickly replace hemp as the fabric of choice for clothing and textiles.   While the consumption and sale of alcohol became illegal during Prohibition in 1919, Americans were initially encouraged to explore marijuana as a safer alternative, however, once the 1937 Marijuana Tax Act was passed by Congress, all forms of cannabis use became a criminal offense.

Interestingly enough, after the United States was attacked by Japan at Pearl Harbor, signaling the beginning of America's involvement in World War Two, it became extremely difficult to import industrial hemp from countries in eastern Asia. Therefore, the industrial production of hemp was once again not only allowed but in fact heavily encouraged by American farmers, particularly in the Midwest. While hemp cultivation was linked with patriotism for this brief period in time, once the war had ended, so did any legal rights to growing hemp in the United States.

In 1951, the Bogs Act and Narcotic Control Act put the final nail in the coffin of industrial hemp production when the United States Government grouped hemp, marijuana and all other forms of cannabis in together as a singular substance, outlawing all forms for their supposed detrimental effect on the mind and body of those who used them for recreational or therapeutic purposes. By 1957, all forms of industrial hemp was banned in the United States.

While the 1970 Comprehensive Drug Abuse Prevention and Control Act allowed for cannabis to be distinguished from other narcotics such as cocaine due to its marked therapeutic benefits, Regan's 1986 Anti-Drug Abuse Act and subsequent War on Drugs called for mandatory criminal sentences for anyone caught possessing or selling drugs, whether it be marijuana, heroin or another substance.

California is credited with being the first state to legalize cannabis when it was permitted in 1996 for medicinal purposes. The Clinton administration, however, was determined to continue the War on Drugs, and many patients were arrested for imbibing in medical marijuana, as were the physicians who prescribed the treatment. It was not until the Obama administration came onto the scene in 2009 that medicinal use of cannabis was decriminalized, though recreational marijuana use was still considered illegal.

In modern times, the leading world producers of hemp are Canada, France, China and Great Britain. It was not until the year 2014 that hemp farming finally became legal again after Barack Obama passed a law allowing for limited hemp cultivation in the United States. Currently, there are twenty-one states that legally permit hemp growing. They are California, Colorado, Delaware, Hawaii, Illinois, Indiana, Kentucky, Maine, Michigan, Missouri, Montana, Nebraska, New York, North Dakota, Oregon, South Carolina, Tennessee, Utah, Vermont, Washington and West Virginia.

Why Grow Hemp?

Some of the major advantages of growing hemp over other crops are as follows:

Hemp is Super-Strong: Hemp is one of the world's strongest natural fibers, being over ten times stronger than other common fabric materials, such as cotton, nylon, silk or wool. This makes is a useful material for making rope, clothing and other durable goods.

Hemp is Very Diverse, and it Saves A lot of Space: Hemp is a hearty plant, and it can withstand a wide range of temperature and soil conditions. This means that is can be grown in most environments and climates, compared to cotton, which cannot withstand the colder temperatures of the North or the drier conditions of the West. Farmers like hemp because they get a higher return on their initial investment. Compared to cotton or flax, hemp plants can thrive even when they are planted very close together. This allows for a much higher yield per acre.

Hemp Gives a lot Per Individual Plant: As deforestation becomes a very serious issue, hemp is very sustainable as well as profitable. A single acre of hemp is capable of producing up to four times more paper than the wood from an acre of trees. Likewise, hemp grows back many times faster than trees, reaching full maturity within four months instead of a span of multiple years. Hemp is unusual in that is does not exhaust the soil it is grown in or strip it of minerals. Rather, hemp seems to enrich the soil it is grown in, meaning that one farmer could conceivably grow three full, healthy hemp crops each year.

Hemp has a Great Deal of Nutritional and Medicinal Value: Hemp seeds are very high in protein, making them a valuable addition to any idea, yet particularly valuable for vegetarians and vegans. The seeds are also very rich in Vitamin E, which means that they not only benefit the skin but help to strengthen the body's natural immune system as well. The oil produced from hemp, known as CBD hemp oil has a multitude of marked health benefits, including providing relief from seizures, preventing strokes, quelling symptoms of ADD/ADHD and relieving anxiety and depression.

How is CBD Hemp Oil Used?

There are a multitude of methods for using CBD oil, both internally and externally which are discussed in their own separate chapter. However, the most common form of using CBD oil is to consume it sub-lingually in a tincture form, meaning that the drops are administered underneath the tongue. CBD oil may also be made into edibles such as cookies, brownies or candy as well as inhaled through a vaporizer, incorporated into a mouth or nose spray and/or made into a topical lotion, balm or salve.

What are the Potential Side-Effects of CBD Hemp Oil?

Due to the legal issues surrounding cannabis, there is a lack of research on CBD hemp oil as well as medical marijuana. Currently, the Food and Drug Administration classifies it as being possibly safe for adult consumption. Generally speaking, CBD oil is mostly considered to be safe for internal and external use amongst many medical and alternative healing communities, yet there are some potential side effects and interactions associated with its use that must be carefully considered before beginning treatment. Some patients report minor ailments, such as sleeplessness, a feeling of light-headedness and/or diminished saliva production. Some patients also experience issues with lowered blood pressure after taking CBD oil as well. Some doctors caution patients to avoid ingesting grapefruit juice while undergoing CBD hemp oil treatment as well.

Patient's with Parkinson's Disease are warned to avoid using CBD hemp oil, as it is theorized that it may actual make tremors and shaking worse. Additionally, it is important that pregnant women abstain from all forms of CBD Hemp oil use as well. Those women who are in the progress of nursing a child should avoid use as well, along with babies and infants. Small children may benefit from low dosages of CBD oil, though it is absolutely vital that the lowest possible effective dose is used, and that the child's progress is monitored by a qualified medical professional.

Chapter Two: Hemp vs Marijuana

Many people mistakenly believe that hemp and marijuana are the same thing. Given the history, it is easy to see why the confusion is so common, seeing that they have often been treated as the same substance by the United States government. While both hemp and marijuana come from the Cannabis plant, there are a multitude of differences between the two. Cannabis itself is one of the oldest domesticated crops in the United States, having been cultivated by such great historical figures as George Washington, John Adams and Thomas Jefferson. In fact, the Declaration of Independence, which is often considered to be the most defining document in American history was printed on paper derived from the cannabis plant!

So what is the difference?

The leaves and flowering tops of the cannabis plant contain what is known as tetrahydrocannabinol, more commonly referred to as THC. These are the only parts of the cannabis plant that contain psychoactive properties, and thus, they are harvested, dried and smoked or made into edibles for their mind-altering and therapeutic effects. THC is what makes a person feel high or "stoned" after smoking or consuming marijuana. The higher the concentration of THC in a particularly cannabis plant, the stronger the psychoactive effect is on the user.

Hemp, on the other hand, comes from the seeds and stalks of the cannabis plant rather than the buds. This part of the plant contains a very miniscule amount of THC, which makes it useless for any kind of recreational drug use. Hemp instead has very highly concentrated levels of something called cannabidiol, which is more commonly referred to as CBD Hemp oil.

Generally speaking, marijuana plants are smaller and bushier than hemp plants. Marijuana is more difficult to grow as well, as it is far fussier than its cousin, relying upon ample sunlight and plenty of growing space to ensure proper flowering and multiple buds. Marijuana farmers are concerned with maximizing THC content and care only about cultivating the buds or flowering tops of the plant, while those growing hemp are concerned with strengthening the cannabis' stalk.

To put the difference between marijuana and hemp into perspective, the average strain of marijuana boasts about fourteen to twenty percent THC. However, in order to classify as hemp instead of marijuana, cannabis must be an absolute maximum of one percent THC, though levels as low as 0.03 percent are standard in Colorado and other states.

Not only is there a big difference between marijuana and hemp, there is also a difference between hemp oil and CBD Hemp oil. Hemp oil is produced solely from the seeds, and acts as a natural demulcent and emollient for the skin. This makes it a popular addition to moisturizers, lip balms, lotions and other cosmetics. CBD Hemp oil, however, is more commonly used for medicinal and/or therapeutic purposes. While hemp oil contains zero THC, CBD Hemp oil does contain trace amounts, **though not enough to stimulate any psychoactive effects.** To reiterate, CBD has no psychoactive properties.

Let's Talk Legalities

Ok, so you're probably wondering if you'll get "high" while taking Hemp Oil or CBD. While the FDA currently groups marijuana and hemp together under the category of cannabis, the simple fact is that hemp contains absolutely zero psychoactive or mind-altering properties.

Therefore no matter how much hemp or CBD Hemp oil a patient consumes or inhales, they will not get high or feel "stoned."

States That Have Legalized Industrial Hemp Production
- Alabama, Arkansas, California, Colorado, Florida, Georgia, Hawaii, Illinois, Indiana, Kentucky, Maine, Michigan, Minnesota, Mississippi, Montana, Nebraska, Nevada, New Hampshire, North Carolina, North Dakota, Oregon, Pennsylvania, Rhode Island, South Carolina, Tennessee, Utah, Vermont, Virginia, Washington and Wyoming.

States That Have Legalized Hemp Oil/CBD Hemp Oil
- Legal in all fifty states, though CBD Hemp oil is still illegal in Idaho, Indiana, Kansas, Nebraska, South Dakota and West Virginia.

States That Have Legalized Medicinal Marijuana

- Alaska, Arizona, Arkansas, California, Colorado, Connecticut, Delaware, Florida, Hawaii, Illinois, Maine, Maryland, Massachusetts, Michigan, Minnesota, Montana, Nevada, New Hampshire, New Jersey, New Mexico, New York, North Dakota, Ohio, Oregon, Pennsylvania, Rhode Island, Vermont, Washington, Washington DC and West Virginia.

States That Have Legalized Recreational Use of Marijuana

- Alaska, California, Colorado, Maine, Massachusetts, Nevada, Oregon and Washington.

Chapter Three: Benefits of Hemp Oil and CBD for Physical Injuries & Ailments

CBD Hemp oil does not contain a high enough level of THC to produce any kind of psychoactive effect on those who use it. Thus, individuals who utilize CBD Hemp oil as a component in a therapeutic regimen will not experience any mind-altering side effects, but will still reap the medicinal benefits.

The human body has an endocannabinoid system which includes receptors all over the body. CBD Hemp oil, like all other cannabinoids attaches itself to these receptors, of which there are two kinds. CBD1 receptors are mostly located in the brain, and these are also the receptors that are most highly affected by the presence of THC. CBD2 receptors are located throughout the entire body, yet rather than being connected with the brain, they are connected to the immune system. CBD Hemp oil works by stimulating the body's CBD2 receptors, helping to fight off and prevent diseases.

CBD Hemp oil has been shown to have a dramatic effect upon a number of physical ailments, such as

Multiple Sclerosis: Commonly referred to as MS, Multiple Sclerosis causes miscommunication in the nerves, meaning that signals between the brain and body are often askew. Patients may suffer from an inability to move their arms or legs, blindness or compromised vision, uncontrollable shaking as well as a feeling of electricity that passes through the neck.
CBD hemp oil is being shown to provide relief to MS patients. It can help reduce pain levels as well as quell body tremors. Multiple sclerosis often interferes with its victims' sleep patterns, and CBD hemp oil can also be useful for promoting sleep.

Recommendation: Multiple sclerosis is best treated with CBD oil strains that carry a high CBD level, such as Charlotte's Web or Sour Tsunami.

Diabetes: Diabetes is a disease which is characterized by the body's inability to produce enough insulin. Insulin production is what regulates the body's blood sugar or glucose level. There are two types of diabetes. In type one diabetics, the body has a problem making insulin, while in those with type two, the body does not properly utilize the insulin it makes.

Over 30 million Americans are diabetic. Complications from the disease can result in neuropathy and nerve damage in the feet and hands as well as damage to the eyes, kidneys and cardiovascular system.

Studies conducted at the Hebrew University of Jerusalem suggest that CBD oil's ability to reduce inflammation may stabilize the metabolism of those who suffer from type two diabetes. Diabetics can also benefit from CBD hemp oil's ability to reduce the neuropathy in the fingertips and toes

There is some research that suggests that using CBD oil can actually prevent diabetes by improving fasting blood sugar levels and combatting obesity, which is one of the leading causes of Type II diabetes. However, there are only limited resources for this topic, so it should strictly be considered a theory at this point in time.

Alzheimer's Disease: Alzheimer's Disease is characterized by the onset of dementia which progresses over time. Symptoms of dementia include confusion, loss in short and long-term memory, changes in mood and difficulty problem solving and /or completing everyday tasks.

Alzheimer's Disease is a terrifying diagnosis. The memory gradually decreases until patients are unable to recognize the people around them. Patients with moderate to advanced Alzheimer's Disease may find themselves suddenly confused as to their location or the period of time they are living in. This can understandably cause these patients to experience moments of panic or aggression towards their surroundings.

There is some research demonstrating that small amounts of THC can slow the production of beta-amyloid proteins, which are a key factor in the progression of the disease. Both the American Journal of Alzheimer's Disease and the Salk Institute have research on this topic. There is also evidence of CBD's usefulness in helping to stabilize the mood swings and wandering that are so characteristic of the illness.

Epilepsy: Epilepsy is a neurological condition that is characterized by the sudden onset of seizures that do not have another underlying cause. In order for a person to be diagnosed as an epileptic, they must have experienced at least two unexplained seizures.

CBD oil can be used to help epileptics control their seizures. While epilepsy cannot be cured, CBD oil is effective at lessening the time and intensity of the convulsive episodes. A 2017 study by the New England Journal of Medicine found a 23% decrease in seizures among child epilepsy patients taking CBD oil when compared to those taking a placebo. In fact, there is evidence that cannabis and its derivatives have been used to treat epilepsy since the 1800s. It is a particularly valuable alternative for doctors who are hesitant to increase the dosage in patients receiving traditional seizure drugs with major side effects.

Cancer: Cancer is basically the renegade mutation of cells in the body. The cancer cells reproduce rapidly and attack healthy cells. There has been a great deal of excitement emerging over the pronounced effect that CBD oil has on these cancer cells. Not only does CBD oil appear to prevent cancer cells from spreading throughout the body, it also attacks active cancer cells.

CBD oil has been shown to improve patient prognosis in a number of cancers, including brain, breast, colon, lung, prostate as well as leukemia. CBD oil is thought of in many circles as being the miracle cure for cancer that doctors and rest of modern medicine has been seeking for years.

Research by the American Association of Cancer Research has shown that Cannabinoids can be useful in the treatment of prostate cancer. A study by the Journal of Neurochemistry on mice found that CBD helped reduced cancer growth rates within test subjects.

Chapter Four: Benefits of Hemp Oil and CBD for Mental Health

Treating mental health disorders is one of the absolute biggest money makers for the pharmaceutical companies. Patients who suffer from anxiety, depression, obsessive-compulsive disorder, manic depression and post-traumatic stress disorder are given a cocktail of different medications which simultaneously dull their symptoms as well as their personalities.

Each separate disorder has a multitude of pills currently available on the market which are geared towards alleviating the symptoms. Aside from causing feelings of general disconnection from the rest of the world and chronic fatigue, many of these medications carry very potentially serious side effects and actually cause dependency upon the medication.

For example, Zoloft and Lexapro are two of the most commonly prescribed medications for treating clinical depression. Depression is a very common mental health disorder which varies in its severity which results from a chemical imbalance in the brain. While the above medications help to correct this imbalance, both also carry with them the risk of causing tremors, agitation and even seizures in their users.

A panic disorder is characterized by the sudden onset of intense fear. These panic attacks may or may not be caused by an external trigger, such as a certain noise or smell. Patients with a pronounced panic disorder can have difficulty completing day to day activities, as their irrational fears may prevent them from engaging in simple tasks, such as socializing with others. Alprazolam and Lorazepam are both proven to help with the symptoms of anxiety, yet these drugs are also extremely addictive, and the patient may quickly build a tolerance to them, leading to a need for an increased dosage. Patients may also suffer from major withdrawal and even death if they are to stop taking these medications suddenly, as the body becomes dependent upon them.

CBD hemp oil is being slowly recognized for its ability to effectively treat many forms of mental illnesses and psychiatric disorders. While it does provide relief for the symptoms patients experience, it is particularly valuable because unlike its Big Pharma counterparts, CBD oil is able to provide results without the risk of major side effects or forming an addiction.

First and foremost, CBD oil is a very powerful anti-psychotic. This means that administering a few drops underneath the tongue of a patient who is undergoing some sort of mental crisis has an almost instantaneously calming, soothing effect, thereby working to de-escalate the initial crisis.

Patients who suffer from schizophrenia often report the presence of auditory and even physical hallucinations. They may hear voices speaking to them in an empty room, or may see the presence of people who are not really there. Schizophrenics are often unable to truly determine what is real and what is a product of the disease, and can become easily agitated, combative or even violent. CBD oil has shown to help decrease these hallucinations as well as to stabilize the mood in patients with schizophrenia. A 2011 study in Schizophrenia Research showed that CBD was associated with significantly lower degrees of psychotic symptoms. The two authors of the study T.A. Iseger and M.G. Bassong went on to conclude that the studies "further confirm the potential of CBD as an effective, safe and well-tolerated antipsychotic compound"

Another mental disorder which benefits from CBD oil is post-traumatic stress disorder. Particularly prevalent amongst veterans and trauma survivors, PTSD is characterized by the sudden onset of flashbacks, in which the patient is transported back in their mind to a traumatic moment in their personal history. For a veteran, they may feel as though they are back on the battlefield after hearing a firework discharge, whereas an abuse survivor may have a flashback triggered by hearing a man yell loudly across the street.

CBD oil has shown promise in helping to reduce the frequency of these flashbacks by lowering the initial anxiety levels in patients with PTSD. Unlike the traditional medications which are usually prescribed for PTSD, CBD oil helps promote a feeling of calm without dulling the other senses.

Chapter Five: Benefits of Hemp Oil and CBD Oil for Learning Problems

It is not only physical and mental illnesses that can be beneficially treated with CBD hemp oil. Studies have shown the drug to be tremendously effective for patients who are diagnosed with a broad spectrum of learning disabilities, including ADD/ADHD and those who fall on the autism spectrum.

ADD (Attention Deficit Disorder) and ADHD (Attention Deficit Hyperactivity Disorder) are commonly diagnosed in children around the age of seven or eight, and symptoms may disappear with age or present themselves throughout a lifetime. ADD/ADHD is a very common disorder which is characterized by an inability to focus and concentrate on the task at hand. Oftentimes, students with ADD/ADHD may seem as though they are constantly fidgeting or otherwise goofing off, yet this is not due to an intentional rebellion but rather the fact that their brains simply handle a lack of stimulation far worse than others. ADD/ADHD students are often highly intelligent, yet they may fall behind in their classes due to an inability to focus long enough to express aptitude in any subject.

People who suffer from ADD/ADHA often have very low levels of dopamine in their brains. As dopamine is the chemical which is responsible for causing feelings of happiness and contentment, these individuals who lack the chemical can suffer from inexplicable bouts of anger and irritability. Hemp oil and CBD help provide increased dopamine to the brain, which helps reduce aggression in ADD/ADHD patients.

Another learning disorder which seems to benefit from CBD hemp oil treatment is autism and Asperger's disease. While many people mistakenly believe they are the same ailment, there are some key differences:

Autism Spectrum Disorders are characterized by issues with communication and socializing. The symptoms of autism vary considerably from one person to another. Those who have a mild case of autism may experience difficulty interacting with others, preferring instead to fixate intently on certain areas of life, such as a particular school subject or hobby. On the more extreme end of the autism spectrum, patients may be completely non-verbal and dependent upon help from others to complete basic day to day tasks, such as dressing, feeding or washing oneself.

Asperger's Disease is a form of high-functioning autism. While many who fall along the autism spectrum experience marked developmental delays, those with Asperger's typically have an IQ that is on par with or superior to their peers. They do, however, experience difficulty with socializing, and may have trouble making eye contact, feeling empathy for others or engage in repetitive actions or movements, such as rocking, counting, moving objects, etc.

CBD oil has been shown to help alleviate some of the most problematic symptoms of autism and Asperger's. Studies including those in Current Neuropharmacology suggest that CBD oil not only helps to alleviate the obsessive tendencies which are common to both disorders, it also decreases levels of anxiety, thus allowing the individual to relax in social situations. CBD oil is also helpful for stabilizing the mood swings and bouts of aggression which can result from frustration at not being able to effectively communicate.

Chapter Six: Benefits of Hemp Oil and CBD Against Aging

The skin is the largest organ on the human body. As we age, the collagen in our skin begins to break down, which leads to wrinkles, fine lines and other signs of aging. There are a multitude of environmental factors which accelerate visible signs of aging in the skin, such as smoking, sun exposure and the pollution levels in the air.

Hemp oil and CBD are incredibly beneficial to the skin. CBD oil is a powerful antioxidant that can combat the effects of aging better that Vitamin E or C. The topical application of hemp oil causes the CBD to be absorbed quickly through the skin cells, as the cannabinoid receptors highly concentrated here. The oil not only helps to protect against the harmful UV rays from the sun, it also forms a shield between the skin and any free radicals that may be present within an environment. A study in Swiss research paper Molecules confirmed CBD's antioxidant and anti-aging properties.

One of the largest factors that contributes to aged skin is a lack of moisture. Hemp oil is a common addition to many salves, balms and lotions for its ability to quench the skin's thirst without leaving behind a residue.

Aside from toll that aging can take on the skin, it can also wreak havoc on maintaining a sleep schedule. Most people need anywhere from six to nine hours of sleep a night, with the need being greater in infancy and less in older age. Disruptions in sleep as well as general insomnia are an unfortunate side effect of getting older, and a consistent lack of sleep can lead to health issues as well as agitation. Hemp oil and CBD is highly effective at promoting a regular sleep cycle in individuals of all ages, yet it is particularly valuable for helping to alleviate insomnia in patients over sixty years old.

Chapter Seven: Benefits of Hemp Oil and CBD for Pets

It is not only humans that reap the benefits of hemp oil and CBD, it has also been proven to have a number of beneficial effects on domestic pets, such as cats and dogs. In recent years, studies have been carried out specifically on dogs to prove the effectiveness of CBD in small doses. Previously, owners were self-dosing dogs and cats with human grade edible marijuana, which is not safe. However, pioneering studies by Veterinarians at Colorado State University have allowed us to determine safe levels of CBD oil for pets. When taken in appropriate dosages (a general rule of thumb is to administer one milligram per ten pounds of body weight), CBD helps alleviate many behavioral problems as well as alleviating symptoms of physical diseases.

How Can Hemp Oil and CBD Help My Pet?

Hemp oil and CBD have a marked calming effect

Some animals are simply higher strung by nature than others. Cats or dogs who have been rescued from an abusive or neglectful situation may suffer from a form of animal post-traumatic stress disorder which causes anxiety and even flashbacks. Even if they have been raised in a loving environment from day one, animals with a nervous temperament are more prone to obsessive tendencies and anxious behavior. This anxiety can manifest in a number of undesirable ways, from chewing/clawing furniture to urinating/defecating in in appropriate areas or even outright biting and scratching.

Even animals that are not prone to anxiety may experience intense fear when exposed to loud noises, such as thunder, gun shots or hammering. Hemp oil and CBD is effective in helping to calm these fears by stimulating the brain's natural supply of cannabinoids. This provides a sense of calmness and an increase in endorphins, which eliminates the feeling of panic and danger.

CBD is valuable for pain management

CBD oil not only helps eliminate nervous energy in dogs and cats, it can also assist with relieving symptoms associated with old age, such as arthritis. CBD oil can combat the inflammation in the joints which causes the pain associated with arthritis, and may also be able to help preserve vision and prevent cataracts.

Animals who undergo surgery can benefit from CBD oil as well, as it helps lower pain levels without affecting respiration or consciousness. Likewise, CBD oil promotes restfulness, which helps provide a serene environment that helps with speeding along the recovery process after an accident or surgery by promoting a calming mindset that emphasizes relaxation and rest. Hemp oil and CBD is also effective at helping to treat physical discomfort associated with cancer and other diseases in domestic dogs and cats.

CBD helps prevent symptoms of aging

A regular regimen of CBD hemp oil helps to prevent against arthritis, stiff joints, loss of appetite, lethargy and other common symptoms of aging in mature dogs and cats. Regular administration of CBD assists with maintaining brain health as well.

Chapter Eight: Benefits of Hemp Oil and CBD for Fibromyalgia

Fibromyalgia is a disease characterized by moderate to intense nerve pain known as neuropathy. This pain can seem to radiate throughout the whole body, though medical tests may show no concrete reason for the discomfort. Patients with fibromyalgia may suffer from what appears to be phantom pain, meaning that there is no viable explanation for what is actually hurting. These pains are often widespread and chronic, occurring over the entire body for up to four months at a time. No one is entirely sure what causes fibromyalgia, though it is markedly more common in women than men. While there is no known cure, patients are able to control their symptoms with a variety of medications.

The most common prescription medications for fibromyalgia are Lyrica, Cymbalta and Neurontin. All of these drugs are certainly effective in relieving the nerve pain associated with fibromyalgia, yet all carry some very serious potential side effects and interactions.

Lyrica: (Pregabalin) Minor side effects include vertigo, dry mouth, limb swelling and weight gain, while serious side effects range from extreme fatigue, blurred vision and even potential major kidney damage. In some patients, Lyrica can cause aggression and suicidal tendencies as well.

Cymbalta: (Duloxetine) Some of Cymbalta's minor side effects are nausea, constipation or fatigue. Like Lyrica, Cymbalta has been known to cause extreme, dangerous mood shifts in some patients which can result in extreme aggression or suicide if not immediately treated. Another potentially serious side effect of Cymbalta is uncontrolled muscle stiffness and/or seizure activity.

Neurontin: (Gabapentin) While Neurontin is most commonly used to control seizure activity in epileptics, it does help to relieve symptoms of fibromyalgia as well. Less serious side effects include fatigue and a lowered immune system, however Neurontin can also uncontrolled eye movement as well as changes in behavior and mood. Some may find that their mood swings are amplified and far more intense, while others may experience severe depression and/or anger.

The commonly prescribed medications for fibromyalgia are valuable in that they certainly provide the patient with relief from the nerve pain which is the hallmark of the disease. However, these drugs all carry with them very serious side effects, most remarkably on the detrimental effect they can have on the patient's mental health.

Hemp oil and CBD have not been proven in any official medical studies to alleviate the pain associated with fibromyalgia, yet there is a large population of patients who are urging the medical community to do more research on this topic. Many victims of fibromyalgia stop taking their medication due to an inability to tolerate the drug's side effects. CBD oil shows remarkable potential for alleviating the symptoms without any of the potentially dangerous psychological side effects.

Chapter Nine: Different Types of Hemp CBD Oil

Hemp Oil

There are two primary forms of hemp oils. Hemp seed oil is either unrefined or refined. Unrefined hemp oil is cold pressed, meaning that there is very minimum heat used when extracting the oil from the cannabis plant, which means that it retains the majority of its nutritional and anti-oxidant properties. Refined hemp oil is nature's equivalent of bleached flour. Virtually all of the nutritional and therapeutic properties have been lost in the refining process, though the oil is still good for topical use, such as making soaps and/or moisturizers.

CBD Hemp Oil

CBD hemp oil is entirely different. It is a cannabinoid that is extracted from the hemp plant. While it affects the cannabinoid receptors in the brain, it does not contain any psychoactive properties, which means that it does not get its users "high", no matter if it is smoked, consumed or applied topically.

Types of CBD Oil

Rick Simpson Oil

One of the most popular forms of CBD oil is Rick Simpson Oil, which was concocted by the medical marijuana pioneer and activist of the same name. After Simpson used this particular concentration of oil to cure himself from skin cancer over ten years ago, he was determined to bring his message of alternative healing to the greater population. Unlike CBD oil, Rick Simpson oil contains THC as well, which can be undesirable for some patients. The Indica strains of Rick Simpson oil are used to treat physical ailments, while sativa strains have proven to work well on patients with anxiety, PTSD and other mental ailments. While the oil is available for purchase online, albeit illegally, those in need of its benefits are able to create the medicine in their own homes by following Simpson's detailed online instructions, as long as all necessary safety precautions are taken. These instructions can be found at www.phoenixtears.ca

High CBD Cannabis Strains

CBD oil is made out of cannabis which contains high levels of CBD rather than THC. This means that while the psychoactive properties are non-existent, the healing properties of the cannabis plant are magnified. The top strains of CBD oil that have the highest levels of CBD are Charlotte's Web, Harlequin, Sour Tsunami and Cannatonic.

Chapter Ten: User Experiences with CBD Oil

CBD oil users of all ages and backgrounds have a forum to share their experiences and suggestions with one another at www.420evaluationsonline.com.

Bi-Polar Disorder

While there is a plethora of first- hand accounts which illustrate the various ways in which CBD oil's valuable healing properties have improved the lives of countless individuals, one of the most moving accounts comes from a young man named Casey who suffers from manic depression, otherwise known as bi-polar disorder. Casey states that he even though he knew he was sick, he refused to go on medicine for years because he was afraid of the potential side effects. While Casey shunned the thought of drugging himself into a stupor with traditional medications, he began doing research on his own, and came across a website that advertised the benefits of utilizing CBD as an alternative to psychotropic drugs.

Casey's mood swings had increased in intensity along with his anxiety to the point where he decided he had nothing to lose by giving CBD oil a try After only two weeks of using CBD oil, he reports a dramatic decrease in his symptoms, to the point where he is able to go to work "for the first time in ten years without having anxiety."

Asperger's Syndrome

A woman named Adrienne reports that she was initially hesitant to explore CBD oil, mistakenly believing that it was the same as marijuana. However, after she continued to read more information, Adrienne and her husband made the decision to purchase CBD oil in an attempt to help their son, who suffers from Asperger's Syndrome, relieve his social anxiety. Adrienne conducted a series of tests, all which proved to her and her family beyond a shadow of a doubt that CBD oil was invaluable for helping their son live his life as normally as possible. For example, Adrienne states that her son fixated on all kinds of sports, and was previously easily thrown into hysterics by any sort of change to his expected routine.

One day, her son got the time wrong for his sport's camp, and instead of becoming agitated and going into a full-blown anxiety attack, he was able to simply place a calm phone call to his mother asking that she come pick him up. It is not only the couple's son that has benefited from CBD oil. Adrienne's husband uses the oil for its ability to relieve digestive issues as well as for nausea and vertigo associated with motion sickness.

Skin Cancer

Of course, no chapter dedicated to CBD oil user's experiences would be complete without discussing Rick Simpson. A film producer who is a major advocate for the legalization of marijuana and all hemp production, his film *Run from the Cure* expresses his dismay at the advantage the pharmaceutical company has over patients with cancer. Simpson in fact claims that CBD oil can be used to cure many forms of carcinoma, as it did with his own skin cancer.

It is not only Rick Simpson who advocates for CBD oil's cancer curing properties. A woman named Sharon Kelly was diagnosed with Stage four small-cell lung cancer which had spread to the lymph nodes and stomach. Her prognosis was considered terminal, and she was given less than a year to live. After all attempts at chemo failed, Kelly's daughter began to research CBD oil on the internet, and was encouraged by what she saw. Figuring that she may be able to buy herself more time, Kelly began using CBD suppositories. Only seven months after beginning daily CBD oil treatment, not only had Kelly's tumors shrunk, they had completely disappeared! Her doctors were absolutely baffled by the fact that she has remained cancer-free for over one year!

Schizophrenia

A teenage girl by the name of Stephanie credits CBD oil with saving her life. Diagnosed as a paranoid schizophrenic at the age of sixteen, Stephanie suffered from regular bouts of intense auditory and sensory hallucinations, where she would hear voices instructing her to hurt herself and the people around her, as well as a pervasive sensation of being scratched, pinched and touched.

Stephanie began receiving intense psychiatric treatment shortly after being diagnosed. In addition to intense therapy, she was prescribed no less than seven different medications to take each day, along with two other PRN meds which were provided in case of a psychotic break or extreme episode.

Stephanie faithfully took her medicine and adhered to her therapy schedule. While the intensity and frequency of her schizophrenic symptoms was alleviated by the medicine, she also experienced a dramatic decrease in energy. She reports that not only was she sleepy and foggy-brained most of the time, she also began to experience a general feeling of isolation from the general world, leading to thoughts of suicide. Stephanie began undergoing CBD oil treatment about five months ago, and reports a dramatic change not only in her symptoms but in her overall quality of life as well. Not only have the hallucinations drastically reduced, she has an increase in energy which allows her to get back out in the world and participate in the activities she had previously shunned. "I still have to take medicine, but its only one pill a day instead of a handful," she says. "The CBD oil is the best thing I could have done. It has literally saved my life."

Further evidence of CBD's effectiveness in treating schizophrenia is evident on the reddit schizophrenia forum. With users citing "CBD made the voices stop" and "I have been using CBD oil ... for a few months now. It works well. For me, the symptoms of schizophrenia are still there, but lessened."

Anorexia

A young woman who suffered from anorexia for over three years finally found relief in CBD oil treatment. Twenty-three year old Katrina states that she began developing an eating disorder back at the tender age of fourteen, when she first auditioned for her high school cheerleading team. "I was told to come back next year after I'd lost ten pounds," Katrina recalls. "I was about five and a half feet tall, and weighed one hundred and fifteen pounds. I was by no mean fat, or even large. But those words stuck in my head for the rest of my life."

Katrina suffered from anorexia and bulimia for the next three years, at one point weighing in at a mere eighty-nine pounds. She began to develop cardiac issues, as well as alopecia and dental issues.

Katrina underwent intense psychotherapy for her eating disorder, yet it is the introduction of CBD oil that she credits with helping her the most. "My aunt had done a lot of research on it," she says. 'And we gave it a try." CBD oil makes it possible for Katrina to concentrate on the pleasures of life rather than living in a constant state of anxiety.

Pain Management

The Washington Post covered a story which illustrated medical marijuana and CBD oil's benefits for athletes, particularly those who formerly played for the NFL. Some retired players, such as Ebenezer Ekuban sustained injuries during the course of their career that left them with chronic aches and pains ranging from moderate to severe. While such conditions can be treated with a range of prescription pain killers, many former athletes are weary of the potential side effects and addictive nature of these drugs.

CBD oil has been proven to be a valuable part of pain prevention in individuals who suffer from sports related injuries. Steve Foley, who played in the league for 7 years is another former NFL player who utilizes CBD oil as a part of his healing regime, both for pain prevention as well as for help with sleep.

Chapter Eleven: How to Use CBD Hemp Oil

CBD hemp oil takes on different forms, depending upon the individual's preference. Generally available for purchase online as well as in state approved cannabis dispensaries, the recommended dosage is listed on the outside of the product. While there is no definitive dosage that is considered ideal, patients who are new to using CBD oil are encouraged to start with a very small dose that is gradually increased in order to find the right dose for the individual. Finding the ideal dose of CBD can be difficult, and requires time and documentation. One may have to gradually increase and subsequently decrease the dose until the desired results are achieved.

CBD oil is most common inhaled or ingested, though there are other methods of administering. Some of the most common methods of using CBD oil are listed below:

Tincture: This means that the CBD oil has been extracted and combined with alcohol as a solvent. CBD hemp oil tinctures are taken orally, usually by placing underneath the tongue, and come with a dropper that helps calculate dosage. It is important to be sure to shake the tincture thoroughly before each use, as natural separation can occur.

Vaporize: CBD oil can be smoked in a vaporizer, though this method is said to be less effective than ingesting it orally. A vaporizer is simply a tool which heats up the oil, causing it to take on a smoke form that is subsequently inhaled.

Concentrate: A concentrate is usually the strongest dosage of CBD currently available on the market. While these concentrates are administered under the tongue in a manner similar to a tincture, and are far more potent, they also lack any outside flavoring, which can cause some to turn away from them. The taste of raw CBD oil is somewhat bitter and not entirely palatable, which is why it is often combined with other more pleasing elements before ingestion.

Capsules: This form works well for people who do not desire to taste any kind of the CBD oil. These gelatin capsules contain anywhere from 5 to 20 milligrams of CBD apiece, thus it is very easy to keep track of the exact amount entering one's system. The precise dosage of capsules allows patients to more accurately adjust their dosage until they are able to find one that works best for them.

Sprays: CBD Hemp Oil sprays typically have the lowest concentration of CBD, and are therefore generally safer for children and the elderly. In addition to being highly portable, the spray is far more convenient for many people than a tincture or concentrate. CBD oil sprays are typically combined with other natural flavors to improve their taste and appeal.

Balms or Salves: Topical use of CBD hemp oil is effective at softening the skin and reducing visible signs of aging along with having the added benefit of relieving pain in the muscles and joints. Overexposure to the sun can cause extreme pain and subdermal damage, and studies have suggested that applying CBD or hemp oil to the exposed area can lessen the intensity of the burn while also preventing against blistering and peeling.

Chapter Twelve: Guide for Buying CBD Hemp Oil

Hemp oil is legal and permitted for use throughout the entirety of the United States. CBD oil however, is a different matter. As mentioned before, there are still six states which consider hemp and CBD to be no different than marijuana, thus it is still classified as an illegal narcotic, even for medical reasons. These are Idaho, South Dakota, Nebraska, Kansas, Indiana and West Virginia.

In the other forty-four states, the use of CBD oil is legal to treat specific medical conditions, such as epilepsy, cancer, schizophrenia, fibromyalgia, ADD/ADHD, Alzheimer's Disease, etc.
While CBD oil can be purchased in state regulated dispensaries in places where medicinal and recreational marijuana has been legalized, those who live in locations which still prohibit cannabis can gain access to CBD oil by utilizing the internet. There is a wide variety of websites offering various strains of CBD oil at a relatively reasonable price. Provided that one is over the age of eighteen, CBD oil can be purchased by anyone online who has a valid credit card or debit card.

Even major distributors such as Wal-Mart, Target and CVS are exploring the hemp oil and CBD market. Some of the most reputable online places for purchasing CBD oil include NuLeaf and Bluebird.

Unfortunately, CBD oil can be relatively expensive, costing up to sixty dollars for 120 ml, and it is important to consider quality over other more budget friendly options. Even though products with a higher cannabidiol content are more expensive, they also work better with a lower dosage, thus making a better investment per gram than oils with lower levels of cannabidiol.

How to Dose CBD Oil

As with anything, if you haven't tried CBD oil before, it's best to start small. The wonderful thing about CBD oil is that it's easy to increase the dosage by a few mg at a time.
The following is a rough guide for CBD dosing for various ailments. Once again, this is a guide and will vary from person to person - so start small

To increase appetite in cancer patients: 2.5 milligrams of THC by mouth with or without 1 mg of CBD for six weeks

To relieve chronic pain: 2.5-20 mg CBD by mouth for an average of 25 days

To treat epilepsy: 200-300 mg of CBD by mouth daily for up to 4.5 months

To treat movement problems associated with Huntington's disease: 10 mg per kilogram of CBD by mouth daily for six weeks

To regulate sleep disorders: 40-160 mg CBD by mouth.

To treat multiple sclerosis symptoms: Cannabis plant extracts containing 2.5-120 milligrams of a THC-CBD combination by mouth daily for 2-15 weeks. A mouth spray might contain 2.7 milligrams of THC and 2.5 milligrams of CBD at doses of 2.5-120 milligram for up to eight weeks. Patients typically use eight sprays within any three hours, with a maximum of 48 sprays in any 24-hour period.

To treat schizophrenia: 40-1,280 mg CBD by mouth daily for up to four weeks

To treat glaucoma: a single CBD dose of 20-40 mg under the tongue. Doses greater than 40 mg may actually increase eye pressure.

Chapter Thirteen: Growing Cannabis and Making Your Own CBD Hemp Oil at Home

In spite of the recent influx in patients utilizing cannabis for medical and mental health reasons, there are only a certain number of states which allow for the private cultivation of cannabis in any form. Be sure to review the beginning pages of this document for more information on where your own state stands on growing cannabis and making CBD oil.

Most states that allow for legalized marijuana also permit people to grow their own cannabis at home, though the exact number of mature plants permitted per person varies from state to state. In places that have only legalized medicinal marijuana, one must have a doctor's prescription to grow or possess cannabis, though in some cases, a "caretaker" can be nominated. This means that someone other than the patient is legally allowed to grow their supply of cannabis for them, even though the caretaker may not have a legal prescription for marijuana.

Those wishing to cultivate cannabis at home must first start with seeds and a grow room. The quality of the seeds determines the quality of the cannabis, so it is advisable to either purchase seeds from a reputable source or use ones that have previously produced a successful crop.

Having an area of the home specifically designated to the growth of cannabis plants ensures that the amount of light and moisture the plants are exposed to during the growth phase is consistent and easy to alter. Likewise, growing indoors helps prevent against environmental obstacles, such as a drastic drop in temperature or hungry insects which may destroy the crop overnight.

Growing cannabis requires that the growing environment be kept just right. Oftentimes, the lights are put on a timer to ensure that each plant does not receive too little or too much sunlight. Likewise, a constant air flow must be present to allow for proper ventilation. The temperature must be regulated as well, and kept between sixty and eighty-five degrees.

Most cannabis growers cultivate marijuana in soil, yet some prefer to work with hydroponics. In this method, the nutrients that would normally be absorbed through the soil instead go directly to the plants roots via osmosis.

Making Your Own CBD Oil at Home

The first step is selecting the marijuana to use for supplying the oil. Usually anywhere from a quarter to a half an ounce is sufficient. The buds from the cannabis must be chopped finely, or shredded in an herb grinder.

The shredded herb is then placed in a sealed glass mason jar with a cup of extra virgin olive oil or coconut oil and gently shaken before heating the mixture in approximately 200 degree water for between three to four hours. The mixture is then left to cool, then heated in the same way again and cooled before being strained through cheesecloth and set aside for use. The concentration of cannabinoids in the solution is increased with each heating/cooling cycle, so the oil can be tailored to individual use and preference.

The resulting CBD oil should be stored in glass jars in a cool, dry place away from direct sunlight. The mixture should keep at maximum potency for approximately four to six months. When considering making your own CBD oil at home, be sure to consult the precise legal status and regulations regarding your particular state.

Conclusion

We have explored just about every aspect of cannabis and hemp in this manuscript. Perhaps no other plant on the planet is as controversial as the cannabis plant. It has been alternately vilified as a dangerous drug in such cult classic movies as Reefer Madness and heralded as a miracle cure for a variety of physical and mental ailments.

The bottom line is that there are some very obvious healing properties associated with cannabis, whether it is in the form of marijuana or CBD hemp oil. In spite of whatever personal feelings one may have against cannabis, the magnitude of its positive effect in medical and therapeutic cases cannot be simply dismissed.

What does the future hold for cannabis? Many states continue to actively campaign for legalized marijuana, especially after seeing proof with other states such as Colorado that recreational legalization not only can work, it generates a great deal of profitable revenue for the state as well.

CBD hemp oil is gaining recognition for its tremendous healing properties. There is absolutely no question that CBD oil helps to treat the symptoms of different diseases as effectively or more than the drugs which are administered by pharmaceutical companies. As cannabis becomes de-mystified and de-vilified by moving into realm of public research and knowledge, we may find that the answer to combatting physical and mental health issues lies in researching what nature has already provided for us rather than trying to synthesize a cure.

Essential Oils: Discover the Drug-Free, Safe & Inexpensive Way to Combat Anxiety & Stress with 20 DIY Recipes

By Lauren Marshall

Introduction

As little as a few decades ago, essential oils were not very popular in mainstream western culture. Although many different cultures throughout history have utilized essential oils for medicinal and spiritual purposes, much of the knowledge regarding their value was lost. Instead, the subject was deemed a new-age fad, relegated to the same territory as astrology, fortune telling and reading auras. It was not until the end of the twenty-first century that we began to see a renewed interest in the subject. Today, aromatherapy is a reputable subject for practice and study, and essential oils are readily available. You can find them not only in specialty stores geared towards natural healing, but also in major drugstore and on line as well!

It may be difficult for those who are unfamiliar with the subject to believe that essential oils and aromatherapy actual have any true healing properties. Yet, even the most skeptical critic cannot deny the how influential our sense of smell is. Certain smells can trigger memories better than any of our other senses, and these smells also have a marked effect on our mood and state of mind. For example, many people associate the smell of fresh cut grass with summertime. Exposure to the scent triggers receptors in the brain that increase happiness and promote a relaxed, carefree feeling, much as we used to experience during the long warm days of our childhood. Likewise, certain smells may carry negative connotations for certain people. As an example, the smell of gasoline may trigger anxiety and even outright panic in people who have been involved in car accidents.

It is not only the way that smells affect our mood and mental state that makes aromatherapy such an interesting discipline. Certain essential oils also carry some very valid healing qualities. Citrus oils are remarkably stimulating and can assist with elevating energy levels while also increasing the immune system. Tea tree oil is excellent for discouraging ticks and biting insects, while peppermint oil discourages mice and spiders from taking up residence in an area. Lavender oil has been proven to drastically reduce the intensity of migraine headaches, while chamomile oil is wonderful for combatting insomnia and night terrors.

Essential oils are also utilized in many different beauty products. For example, even the most exclusive, pricy designer perfumes are basically composed of one or more essential oils which have been diluted with water. Likewise, a huge amount of personal care items ranging from very expensive to remarkably cheap use essential oils for fragrance and therapeutic benefits. These include soaps, lotions, shampoos, bath bombs, etc. Some companies elect to use fragrance oils instead of essential oils, which means the consumer receives the aromatic smell of the plant but reaps none of the healing benefits.

Historically, essential oils were used out of sheer practicality as well as for their value in medicine, ceremony and spiritual areas. In the days before we had access to flush toilets, running water, refrigeration and other modern conveniences, living conditions were often less than sanitary. Human waste was collected in chamber pots and tossed out into the street, and as there was no garbage man who made the rounds weekly, rotting produce and other waste was often left in the streets to fester. In some areas that were particularly hard hit with plague and other diseases, corpses could be left in piles before they were able to be buried in a mass grave or burned. As one might expect, the result was a powerfully unpleasant smell that permeated the air, as well as an infestation of fleas, rats and other pests running rampant, leading to prime conditions for the farther spread of disease.
Essential oils were not only valued for their ability to cover up the worst of the horrific smell, some were also used for their anti-septic and anti-biotic qualities, as well as for their ability to keep disease spreading pests at bay.

In modern times, we utilize essential oils for cosmetic reasons as well as for the benefits they provide for the mind, body and soul. While essential oils are readily available and anyone can choose to purchase and work with them, it is very important to have a basic working knowledge as to what essential oils are, and what they can and cannot do before beginning to use them. There are definite risks and potentially negative side effects which can occur if you carelessly experiment without knowing what you are doing. As we will discuss more in depth later on, the essential oil market is not very well regulated. In fact, the Food and Drug Administration does not even have a precise definition for essential oils, instead treating them exactly the same as the plant source they came from. The FDA also does not distinguish between essential oils and fragrance oils, so it is very important to know exactly what you are looking for and read the labels before making a purchase. The way that companies advertise is not heavily regulated either. This means that manufacturers can put labels on their bottles which sound appealing and make them stand out from other selections, yet in reality, the terms they use don't really mean anything at all.

The aim of this book is to provide the reader with a basic introduction to essential oils and aromatherapy. Here, you will learn about the benefits as well as the potential risks associated with certain oils, as well as exploring the most popular oils available for purchase today. You will even learn how to create your own essential oil blends to tailor them to your exact need, as well as receiving instruction on how to properly store them for maximum longevity.

Essential oils are wonderful to experiment with once you know what you are doing, so be sure to take the time to educate yourself about each and every oil you choose to utilize. This book will provide you with a basic overview, yet it is necessary to keep in mind that there may be potential risks associated with particular oils that are not specifically covered here. In regards to children and animals, it is always better to be safe than sorry and store the essential oils well out of reach. If your are pregnant or nursing, be sure to consult with your doctor before using any kind of essential oil internally, externally or aromatically.

An Overview of Essential Oils

So what exactly are essential oils? This is a question that can be very confusing for someone who is just beginning to explore the subject, as there is no precise definition. The best way to describe an essential oil is to say that it is a super-concentrated form of a specific plant. Each and every plant contains natural oils within it. These natural oils are in place to create a natural barrier against potential predators and diseases. Because these oils protect the plant, they are necessary, or essential to the vitality of the plant's life. As long the oils are in place, the plant generally remains healthy and unharmed. These oils are found in the plant's blossoms, leaves, bark, resin and roots, and they constitute the major component of essential oils.

When you pick a lavender blossom, you can certainly inhale the scent and derive some of the plant's aromatic gifts. However, a small bottle of lavender essential oil is the end the result of a significant amount of the blossoms which have been condensed into a singular, powerful oil. In the process of becoming an essential oil, everything that is not therapeutic has been removed from the lavender, leaving you only with the parts that have medicinal and spiritual value. Essential oils are far more potent than a plant in its natural form. In fact, many times, a singular drop is enough to produce results! Peppermint oil is another good example. While you can certainly gather fresh or dried peppermint leaves and leave them in the corners of your home to discourage mice and spiders, you can achieve even better results with just a drop or two of the essential oil on a cotton ball!

When you look at a cedar tree, it is difficult to understand how that giant tree could possibly wind up in a small bottle that can be carried around in the pocket. The process of extracting essential oils from the raw plants is something that typically occurs via two different methods – steam distillation and mechanical expression.

Steam distillations uses super-heated steam to release the oils from their protective sacs within the plant. The heat from the steam forces its way through the tiny pores in the plant and collects the oils with it as it passes through. The steam turns into water in a condensation chamber, and the oils rise to the top of the mixture, allowing for easy collection.

Mechanical expression, on the other hand, uses gravity rather than heat for extraction. Essential oils that are obtained via mechanical expression rather than steam distillation may also be referred to as cold pressed. Instead of collection the oils via the use of extreme temperatures, they are instead literally pressed out of the plant via the use of tremendous force and gravitational pull.

The vast majority of essential oils you can find available for purchase are obtained via steam distillation. While this is by far the more common of the two extraction methods, the exception to the rule is in regards to essential oils which are obtained from citrus fruit. Wild orange, grapefruit, lemon and lime oils are all derived via mechanical expression, as the oil comes from applying force to the rind rather than any part of the plant that could be easily distilled.

Some Essential Oil Terminology

Particularly when you are just beginning to learn about and work with essential oils, choosing the right ones can be confusing at best and completely overwhelming at worst. There are a number of different brands and varieties to choose from, and it is very important to be aware that some of these companies will intentionally try to market their essential oils with clever wording and flashy labels to make their product appear to be superior to the competition.

In the process of exploring your choices, you may come across certain bottles of essential oils which carry a label which reads "therapeutic grade." Although the terminology sounds good and may even initially convince you that this particular oil choice is stronger, purer or more valuable for health benefits and aromatherapy purposes, the reality is that the therapeutic grade label means absolutely nothing. This is certainly not to say that the essential oil in question is inferior to other products, it just means that it is not necessarily any better either.

There is no precise or defined set of guidelines in place that deals with regulating different grades and qualities of essential oils. In fact, there is very little regulation in place regarding essential oils in general, as the FDA labels them both a cosmetic and a drug and makes decisions on a case by case basis. As there is no true regulation, the term therapeutic grade is rendered null and void, as any company can elect to use that wording, regardless of their qualifications. It is simply a label that is freely put on the bottle to make the product appear more attractive to the customer rather than a term that carries any kind of true significance.

You will also come across essential oils that are labeled pure vs blended. Here, those two terms definitely do mean two separate and distinct products, and the difference is exactly what it sounds like. An essential oil that is labeled one hundred percent pure means that that bottle of oil contains the oils of only one plant species, while a blend is made up of anywhere from one to many different essential oils. For example, if you are exploring essential oils to assist with a lack of energy, you may elect to purchase a bottle of one essential oil that carries a strong reputation for increasing vitality, such as peppermint, lemon or eucalyptus. However, you may also choose to purchase a pre-blended bottle of oil that contains all three of these individual oils which is specifically geared towards combatting lethargy.

So, is it better to work with pure essential oils, or blended oils? As with everything, there are distinct advantages and setbacks associated with both.

Pure oils are nice to work with because you know exactly what you are getting every time. If you are electing to utilize an essential oil for a particular need, it is important to use a product that contains that oil and that oil only. For example, tea tree oil is very beneficial for the skin, and has the ability to repel insects and ticks. This makes tea tree oil an ideal choice for hikers and those who spend a lot of time outdoors. Pure tea tree oil can be applied to the skin and generally tolerated without any major irritation, however, if you were to apply a blend of tea tree and lemon to your skin, the risks of obtaining a severe sunburn are substantial, as the addition of lemon oil results in heightened photosensitivity.

Anyone who crafts their own essential oil blends must begin with pure oils as a basic stepping stone. If you buy a bottle of pure lavender oil, you can build your own blends precisely to achieve the results you want, whereas if you are trying to work with a lavender blend, there are variables in your recipe that you may be unaware of. Unless you have created the blended oil yourself, it is virtually impossible to be confident of the exact contents.

Blended oils certainly have their advantages as well. While some people may take great delight in concocting their own special blends, others may be interested in utilizing essential oils, but do not have the time or finances to explore each oil individually. Instead of purchasing three or four separate oils and blending them together in precise proportions, it is far more convenient to buy one professionally preblended oil that is specifically geared towards a specific purpose, such as alleviating anxiety or promoting focus and concentration. Those with a busy, on-the-go lifestyle are particularly drawn to essential oil blends, as they can simply place a few drops of one oil into their diffuser and walk away rather than concocting a specialized formula each day.

Aside from convenience, blended oils tend to have the financial edge. Pure essential oils require a large number of raw plant material to produce a small amount of oil. The extraction process can be quite tedious and long, which is why some essential oils, such as neroli and tuberose are extremely expensive in their pure form yet become significantly more affordable when added to a blend.

Essential Oils Vs Fragrance Oils and Perfumes

It can be very confusing to try and distinguish the key difference essential oils and fragrance oils. While some may presume that essential oils are what give a scented candle or air freshener its appealing smell, this is not always true. Oftentimes, these products obtain their scent from synthetic fragrance oils rather than essential oils, which means that the aroma is created in a laboratory rather than in nature. This is the primary difference between essential oils and fragrance oils – one is one hundred percent natural, while the other is not. As a result, the scent you will obtain from product which incorporates lavender fragrance oil may smell exactly the same as products which utilize pure lavender oil, yet in contrast to the pure form, the synthetic version will supply zero health or therapeutic benefits. A bar of soap containing actual lavender oil will not only soften the skin and sooth sunburn, it will contribute a sense of tranquility to the bathing process as well. While lavender soaps scented with synthetic fragrance oils may still provide the appealing smell, the therapeutic benefits do not exist.

Perfumes are created in a laboratory while essential oils are created by mother nature. Synthetic perfume oils serve one purpose, and one purpose only. This is to create a smell which appealing to the human nose. Some designer labels demand upwards of hundreds of dollars for a small bottle of their signature perfume, yet in making this purchase, the customer is paying for sheer smell alone. There are absolutely zero therapeutic benefits associated with even the priciest, most exclusive synthetic fragrance. Even though these companies may advertise that they contain beneficial scents, such as jasmine, lavender or ylang-ylang, these scents are not derived from a natural source, meaning they are not the same.

Not only do synthetic perfume oils tend to be far more expensive than essential oil blends with a similar fragrance, the perfume oil scent is diluted with water or alcohol. Not only does this mean that the fragrance will evaporate from the skin in much less time, it also can leave the skin dried out and irritated from the alcohol.

Essential oils can be applied to the pulse points of the body, such as the inner wrists, inside of the knees and along the throat one time per day, and the scent will continue to be noticeable. Because the oil is super-concentrated rather than diluted, it is long lasting. This means that you not only have to apply your fragrance less often, it means that you use less product, which ultimately saves on money.

Some people have respiratory issues and/or allergies that result in an extreme adverse reaction to synthetic perfume oils. These same individuals are also usually able to tolerate using essential oils, as the natural compounds are not as irritating to the lungs as the synthetic product. This is particularly true in the case of scented candles, air fresheners and other products that rely upon synthetic perfume oils rather than essential oils for fragrance. Not only do these products not carry any therapeutic benefits, even though their label may imply otherwise, they may actually cause harm, as they are essentially diffusing chemicals throughout the area they are used in.

It does bear mentioning that many essential oils are extremely irritating to the skin when applied directly out of the bottle. It is therefore always necessary to utilize a good, quality carrier oil (more on this later) to help create a boundary between the essential oil and the skin. It is also a good idea to do your research beforehand regarding any oil you plan on using. Some essential oils, such as orange, lemon and cinnamon are extremely reactive to sunlight, so you definitely don't want to be wearing them if you're planning on spending the day at the beach or hitting up the tanning bed. As a general precaution, it is always wise to do an allergy/irritant spot test on a very small area of skin before working with the oil.

Essential Oils Throughout History

China: Nature and the natural world has always figured heavily into traditional Chinese medicine; therefore, it comes as no surprise that China is currently one of the biggest exporters of essential oils in the entire world! Chinese medicine uses essential oils for therapeutic ailments. Traditionally, Chinese aromatherapy involves the combination of three separate fragrances, which serve as a top, base and middle note. The top, or high note is intended to disappear quickly, while the middle notes last around eight hours. The base note, however, is the most enduring, in some cases lasting up to two days! Three separate oils may be combined to combat a psychological, spiritual or physical ailment, or simply one may be used, depending upon the situation. For example, a simple top note of something citrus, such as lemon or orange may be all that is needed to restore vitality, while those with chronic fatigue may require the three-fold blend, consisting of a citrus top note and longer acting middle and base notes.

In Chinese culture, any essential oil is believed to be infused with the essence or raw life force of the plant it came from. This essence is called *jing*, and it is a very powerful component in achieving balance between the heart, mind, body and soul as well as for healing a variety of physical and mental ailments. Essential oils are frequently used in conjunction with acupuncture, another ancient form of Chinese medicine that involves stimulating various areas of the body via the insertion of tiny, thin needles.

Egypt: Research shows that essential oils were being used in Egypt as early as 4500 BC! In fact, during ancient Egypt's heyday, you had to be a priest or someone of tremendous spiritual significance in order to work firsthand with essential oils. These oils were considered to be gifts from the gods, and they were therefore too valuable and too sacred to be entrusted in the hands of everyday people. Thus, they were given to those who were seen as being closet to the Gods. The priests were educated in the subject and could distribute the oils accordingly to those who they determined were in need of them, yet they alone had the privilege and/or knowledge of mixing and storing the oils.

The ancient Egyptians were a deeply spiritual culture. They attributed magical qualities to everything from certain animals, such as cats and crocodiles to various plants that were used for ceremonial purposes as well as healing. The ancient Egyptians are responsible for the creation of Kyphi, a blend of over sixteen essential oils that was used in the temples for its extreme spiritual value. Various deities, such as Bastet, Ra and Osiris had their own sacred essential oil blends which were used in ceremony to invoke their favor by anointing their statues. Each Pharo was considered to be an embodiment of the divine, thus they all had their own select blends of oils which were specifically created for them by the priests. These oils were used for many different purposes, depending upon the need at the time. Some would use their oil blend to anoint their weapons before going into battle with the enemy, while others would sprinkle the oil upon their bedsheets to improve their virility and to encourage healthy heirs.

The benefits of essential oils were not only limited to the priests and pharos, however. Cleopatra herself was said to be a huge fan of essential oils from a very young age. She reportedly had a number of blends crafted for her which she regularly used for everything from enhancing her legendary beauty to seducing potential suitors to granting protection from the evil eye.

Greek/Roman: Ancient Greek/Roman culture heavily incorporated essential oils into their everyday lives as well as utilizing them for ceremonial and other spiritual purposes. Certain blends were used to anoint and perfume the body to grant protection and increase bravery before going into battle, while other oils were incorporated into massages and baths to promote relaxation and to increase morale.

Hippocrates was an ancient Greek physician who lived from 460 – 370 BC. If you're not already familiar with his work, he was often referred to as the Father of Modern Medicine, each and every physician must agree to abide by the Hippocratic Oath before commencing practice, meaning that they agree to adhere to a basic code of ethical conduct when they agree to take on the title of doctor. Hippocrates was a strong advocate for aromatherapy or using essential oils for a therapeutic purpose. In order to live a long, healthy live, he believed that every person should indulge daily in an aromatic bath followed by a rigorous massage which also incorporated essential oils.

It is believed that the Greeks were one of the first cultures to begin documenting written knowledge of essential oils, though most of this knowledge was taken from Egyptian culture.

India: The form of healing that was practiced in ancient India is typically referred to as Ayurveda. Ayurvedic medicine is one of the oldest documented medicinal systems in the entire world, originating sometime well over three thousand years ago! The system is centered around the concept of chakras, which are particular areas in the body where energy tends to concentrate. Different essential oils are known to have an effect on different chakras, making them a valuable addition to reiki, meditation and other practices which rely upon balancing the energy of a person's chakras.

- **The Root Chakra:** Located at the base of the spine, this is the chakra that rules over our basic sense of security and belonging in the world. Root chakra work responds to essential oils that are grounding and earth-based in nature, such as patchouli or myrrh.

- **The Sacral Chakra:** Located just below the belly button, this is the chakra that rules over our sense of sexuality, sensuality, passion and creativity. The sacral chakra responds to essential oils that have an aphrodisiac, libido enhancing quality, such as ylang-ylang and sandalwood.

- **The Solar Plexus Chakra:** This is the warrior chakra, the part of our body that determines energy, self-esteem and confidence in our interactions with the world. Working with this chakra requires the ability to honest evaluate oneself, as one may need more cooling or heating oils, depending upon the state of being. For example, if you are a person who tend to have difficulty speaking up for yourself, you may want to concentrate on more stimulating, fiery oils such as cinnamon or black pepper while those who have trouble keeping their tempers in check may benefit from a more soothing, cooling oil such as wintergreen or eucalyptus. Both oils stimulate the chakra, just in a different way.

- **The Heart Chakra:** Located at the heart, this is the center of emotion in the body. Stimulating the heart chakra promotes romance and a relief from anxiety and depression, while the solar plexus chakra regulates the sexual aspects of a relationship. The heart chakra is what binds us to the people we love, as well as that which gives us the strength to endure uncomfortable emotions, such as fear and depression. The heart chakra is affected by essential oils which promote romance and an overall sense of well-being, such as rose and geranium.

- **The Throat Chakra:** The throat chakra, as one would expect, is located in the center of the throat. This chakra rules over our ability to express ourselves and may require attention anytime we feel as though we are afraid to speak up for ourselves, or on the other end of the spectrum, anytime we find ourselves being untruthful or intentionally manipulating others with our words. Healthwise, this is the chakra that has a direct effect on the respiratory system, so those who smoke or experience allergies may find themselves to be particularly benefitted by working with essential oils geared towards this area. The most common essential oils for the throat chakra are mentholated in nature, meaning that peppermint, eucalyptus, wintergreen, spearmint, etc. are often the top choices.

- **The Third Eye Chakra:** Located in the center of the forehead, the third eye chakra is associated with clairvoyance and the ability to perceive and move through the boundaries between our world and spiritual realms. Essential oils associated with the third eye chakra, such as juniper, clary sage and heliotrope are meant to increase our receptivity to spiritual energies while removing psychic and mental blockages. The third eye chakra is a particularly beneficial spot for treating restlessness, attention deficient disorder or even the simple inability to focus and concentrate.

- **The Crown Chakra:** Located at the very top of the head, the crown chakra is our gateway to heaven, the communication point between us on earth and the divine realm. This is the chakra that controls our sense of spirituality as well as that which assists us with delving into mysterious realms, such as clairvoyance, etc. The essential oils which are associated with the crown chakra are those that establish a kind of hot-line between our realm and the otherworld, such as frankincense and elemi.

Aromatherapy

The National Association for Holistic Aromatherapy defines aromatherapy as an "art and science of utilizing naturally extracted aromatic essences from plants to balance, harmonize and promote the health of mind, body and spirit." Simply put, the aromatherapy is the practice of using essential oils to alter ones physical, mental or emotional state of mind.

Before we get into depth about different essential oils and their individual uses, it is important to understand how essential oils are used in aromatherapy in the first place. There are three primary methods of delivering essential oils to the body. These include inhalation, topical absorption and internal ingestion.

Internal ingestion is by far the most controversial and risky method of using essential oils. While some people think nothing of putting a drop of lemon oil in their daily water bottle, it is important to be aware that very few essential oils have actually been deemed safe for internal use. The bottom line is that the research simply isn't there, therefore the long-term risks are unknown. Unless it is absolutely known to be safe, internal use of essential oils is discouraged, particularly in the cases of children or nursing and/or pregnant women. While it is certainly possible for experts to reap the internal benefits of consuming essential oils, there are far less risky and invasive methods that deliver substantial results, as we will discuss below.

The two most common methods of utilizing essential oils lies in topical or aromatic use. Topical use means that the essential oil is applied to the skin, while aromatic use means that the scent is inhaled via a diffuser or simply worn as a perfume for its aromatic benefits.

Many essential oils are beneficial to the skin in a number of ways. Tea Tree oil, for example, can be applied directly to the skin to ward against ticks, mosquitoes, black flies as well as guarding against funguses like athlete's foot and other contagious conditions. Lavender is particularly soothing to the skin and acts as a natural anti-microbial and demulcent, working to regenerate damaged skin cells and minimizing damage from scalds, burns and overexposure to the sun.

Other essential oils have beneficial topical properties, yet they are too powerful in their concentrated form to be applied directly to the skin. This is where the concept of a carrier oil comes into play. Selecting a good quality carrier oil is essential in the practice of aromatherapy, as the carrier oil is what creates a protective boundary between the concentrated essential oil and one's bare skin. Oftentimes, the most popular carrier oils, such as coconut, jojoba, almond, olive and/or Argon oil carry skin-enhancing benefits by themselves as well, including demulcent and emollient properties.

A number of essential oils are highly valued for their ability to repel insects and ticks. Many of these, such as tea tree, peppermint, juniper and eucalyptus can be freely applied to the skin as long as they are diluted in water first. While more information can be found in the essential oil recipe section, a general rule of thumb is to add anywhere from 10 – 20 drops of essential oil to two tablespoons of carrier oil. Likewise, a lightweight, emergency bug spray that is far gentler for children involves a simple 10 drops of essential oil combined with two cups of water and sprayed on exposed areas of the skin as well as on clothing.

By far, the most popular method of using essential oils in aromatherapy is, as one would expect, aromatically. This means that you are directly inhaling the fragrance from the essential oil in order to access its therapeutic and/or spiritual properties. The most common method of delivering essential oils in an aromatherapeutic environment is via a diffuser. Diffusers are an all-natural counterpart to scented candles, and they carry far more health benefits and less risks with them as well.

Some diffusers are made out of rods dipped in essential oil which travels up the rod and diffuses the scent throughout the room, though the most common and potent diffusers are made out of a small glass bowl that is filled with water and five drops of a particular essential oil before being placed above a burning tea light candle. The heat from the candle heats the water and oil, diffusing the scent throughout the area. Other methods include adding drops of oil to bath water or incorporating them into a massage.

While aromatic use is by far the safest way to work with essential oils, it is still not entirely without its risks. Particularly if you are nursing or pregnant, be sure to consult your doctor before using essential oils in any form and keep them well out of the reach of children and animals.

The Most Popular Essential Oils

1. **Angelica:** Angelica oil is derived via steam distillation of the seeds. It is a wonderful essential oil for increasing levels of energy, concentration and overall alertness. Diffuse a few drops of the oil throughout a room while studying or reading for increased clarity and focus, as well as for an overall boost in creativity and inspiration!

   Angelica oil is also wonderful for combatting feelings of lethargy and a lack of energy associated with depression and/or anxiety. It can also assist with relieving respiratory issues as well as with lessening the severity and frequency of migraine headaches.
   Pregnant and/or nursing women should avoid angelica oil in all forms, as it can be toxic to the baby.

2. **Basil:** Basil oil is associated with drawing good luck and prosperity to a home. A few drops of oil diffused throughout an area will help to increase money flow, while inhaling the oil on a regular basis is also believed to stimulate the mood, increase energy levels and promote an overall sense of joy.

   Basil oil is also wonderful for alleviating migraine headaches as well as for encouraging the appetite. It is an effective anti-emetic as well, meaning that it can soothe nausea and upset stomachs.

   Basil oil should never be used internally, as it can be toxic and even fatal in the wrong doses.

3. **Bergamot:** Generally obtained via mechanical expression, bergamot promotes a general sense of well-being, joyfulness and child-like gratitude for the moment at hand. This makes it valuable essential oil for those battling depression and anxiety, as well as for anyone with a generalized sense of overwhelming stress.

   On a physical level, bergamot oil has helped with liver and spleen ailments, as well as encouraging the appetite.

It is however, very important to be aware that bergamot oil is very photosensitive. This means that is can cause irritation to the skin by itself if it is applied with no carrier oil, yet even when the best precautions are taken, it does not react well with direct sunlight. If you are planning on spending time in the sunshine, avoid applying bergamot oil to the skin for at least twenty-four hours before exposure, as severe burns and even blistering can result!

4. **Cedar:** Cedar bark was burned by Native Americans for its ability to purify the spirit and to promote divine protection, and it is used for much the same purposes in modern aromatherapy. Cedar is a scent that is considered to be particularly sacred to the Gods, thus its aroma is believed to ward against all kinds of evil, including repelling diseases and residual negative energy. Adding a few drops of cedar oil to the corners of a home will cleanse the area of any harmful energies that may be lurking, making this a particularly powerful oil for anyone in need of psychic protection. Cedar oil is also wonderful for improving mental clarity along with promoting wisdom and spiritual awareness.
Medicinally, cedar is a wonderful remedy for mild respirator ailments, such as bronchitis or seasonal allergies.

Cedar oil is best used aromatically. It can be toxic in some individuals even when ingested in small doses, and it is very irritating to the skin when used topically. Pregnant women should avoid all forms of use of cedar oil.

5. **Chamomile:** Obtained from the steam distillation of the blossoms, chamomile is well-known for its sedative, calming qualities. The oil can be diffused throughout a room to promote restfulness and to guard against nightmares, while applying it topically works to repel insects. According to some folk legends, chamomile oil is considered very lucky, and can attract wealth and good fortune to anyone who anoints themselves with the oil. Washing your hands in a cup of water that has been mixed with ten drops of chamomile oil is said to encourage monetary flow and professional success, while the oil itself can be used to combat acne, bruising and other skin ailments.

It is interesting to note that those who experience an allergic reaction to ragweed tend to have adverse reactions to using chamomile oil aromatically, so be sure to educate yourself about the potential risks before use. Chamomile oil is not safe for internal use, and any form of ingestion should be avoided unless you are an expert.

6. **Cinnamon:** Cinnamon oil is a very powerful, active essential oil with a number of potent properties. First, it is invigorating, serving to increase alertness and levels of energy. It is considered a very lucky oil as well, working to draw money and prosperity towards anyone who works with the scent. Cinnamon oil not only boosts creativity and overall stamina, it is extremely useful in elevating passion on all levels. This means that it not only increases the libido and draws romantic energy, it can also assist with improving levels of self-confidence and combatting shyness, indifference and/or introversion. Cinnamon oil is very active, which means that it helps to provide speed and intensity to any other oil it is coupled with. This makes it a very potent addition to essential oil blends which are intended to draw love or money.
On a physical level, cinnamon oil helps to strengthen the immune system, and stimulates circulation.

7. **Eucalyptus:** Eucalyptus oil has a powerful, distinctive odor. It is a wonderful oil for students, as it promotes concentration and increases mental clarity. A few drops of eucalyptus oil diffused throughout a room while studying helps with retaining information, as well as with eliminating outside distractions.

Medicinally, eucalyptus oil is a highly effective respiratory aid. It can also be used as a febrifuge, meaning it can combat fevers by lowering the body temperature when the oil is applied to the chest area. Eucalyptus oil has also shown to be an effective remedy against migraine headaches. It is important to note that eucalyptus oil should not be used in any form by those with epilepsy or other convulsive disorders, as it can trigger a seizure. Likewise, women who are pregnant should avoid internal, topical and aromatic use as well. For any individual, internal use of eucalyptus oil is discouraged, as it can be fatal in the wrong doses.

8. **Frankincense:** Frankincense is very soothing, helping to alleviate anxiety and depression while promoting an overall increase in tranquility. If you ever find yourself in a period of extreme stress, add a few drops of frankincense oil to your bathwater and soak for twenty minutes while visualizing all of your negative emotions melting away. A few drops of frankincense oil on the pillowcase will ensure a restful night's sleep, while also increasing sexual energy.

   On a physical level, frankincense is excellent at boosting the immune system, and can be used to keep all forms of sickness at bay! As the oil naturally repels germs, it is a popular natural remedy for alleviating dental issues, such as gum inflammation and gingivitis when mixed with water and used as a mouthwash

9. **Ginger:** Ginger is one of the most versatile, valuable essential oils on the market today. It is powerful and stimulating in nature, meaning that it is wonderful for increasing the libido and overall energy levels while promoting happiness, confidence and an overall sense of self-empowerment!

   Ginger oil dramatically improves blood circulation when incorporated into a bath or massage. However, one of the most widely renowned properties of ginger is its ability to soothe nausea and prevent motion sickness. A few drops of the essential oil can be placed on a cotton ball an inhaled for this effect, while a drop or two in a mug of hot water will serve the same purpose. While many pregnant women are able to safely combat the effects of morning sickness by drinking ginger tea or eating small amounts of candied ginger root, it is vital to consult with a doctor before consuming the oil internally if you are pregnant or nursing.

10. **Jasmine:** Jasmine oil is highly beneficial for alleviating stress. Its calming fragrance eases anxiety and banishes depression, making this a highly effective treatment for those who battle with inner demons. A few drops of the oil added to one's pillowcase helps to promote a restful sleep, while wearing the oil topically or adding it to the bathwater is said to assist with drawing romantic energy towards oneself while increasing the libido.

Jasmine oil is good for improving mild respiratory ailments. It is also highly effective at treating issues related to female menstruation, such as helping to alleviate cramping. Some midwives swear by diffusing jasmine oil throughout a room as a woman is giving birth to ease labor pains. Although it is non-toxic and one of the safer oils in general, women who are pregnant or nursing should still avoid all forms of use.

11. **Lavender:** Lavender is perhaps the most popular essential oil in the world. It is widely renowned for its multitude of healing properties, both in regards to the mind and the body. Lavender is extremely soothing; therefore, it helps to promote a calm, tranquil environment. Diffusing lavender throughout a room will help to combat stress while promoting a general sense of well-being.

Lavender promotes restfulness; therefore, it is highly effective in treating cases of insomnia. For children who suffer from night terrors, a few drops of lavender oil on the pillowcase will help to ensure a relief from nightmares while promoting relaxation at the same time. A few drops of the oil can be added to bathwater or simply placed on a cotton ball and inhaled to guard against migraine headaches as well.

Perhaps one of lavender's most valuable healing properties is in regards to its amazing ability to treat burns and scalds. A few drops of lavender oil applied to the affected as soon as possible after burning helps to not only reduce the pain and prevent against blistering, it dramatically speeds up the healing process as well. This healing quality is so marked that many people keep a small bottle of lavender oil in their kitchen specifically for this purpose!

12. **Lemon:** Lemon oil is uplifting by nature. The oil helps to stabilize mood swings by promoting an overall sense of happiness while increasing levels of vitality and energy. Lemon oil can also assist with improving concentration and maintaining focus.

Add a few drops of lemon oil to water for a powerful, all-natural cleaning agent that will fill your house with a delightful fragrance. Lemon oil is a natural anti-biotic, which means that it can help to prevent against disease and illnesses. Adding the oil to one's bathwater is a simple, easy way to boost the immune system, while diffusing the scent throughout the home helps to promote an overall sense of good health and well-being.

As with other citrus oils, lemon oil is extremely photosensitive. This means that you should never wear lemon oil if you are planning on spending any time in the sun. Even without exposure to sunlight, lemon oil can be very irritating to the skin, so be sure to use a quality carrier oil and conduct a spot test before applying in any sort of volume.

13. **Marjoram:** Marjoram oil is highly effective at alleviating anxiety while promoting a sense of calm and tranquility. If you are feeling overwhelmed by stress, adding a few drops of marjoram oil to your bathwater will quiet your mind almost instantly, making this a very effective remedy for over-excited children or those who suffer from mania, obsessive compulsive disorder, etc.

Medicinally, marjoram oil serves as a gentle digestive aid, helping to relieve constipation as well as soothing menstrual cramping. It can also help with alleviating mild respiratory issues and increases circulation when incorporated into massage.

14. **Patchouli:** A grounding essential oil that is linked with stability and nature, patchouli oil is widely revered for its ability to increase the libido amongst both men and women. A particularly valuable essential oil for those who find themselves hindered by sexual inhibitions, diffusing patchouli throughout the bedroom or sprinkling it on the bedsheets helps to alleviate any negative baggage one may carry regarding sex, thus encouraging an enjoyable experience for both partners.

Patchouli oil is also excellent for treating a number of skin conditions. It repels bacteria, acts as an anti-fungal and discourages ticks, mosquitoes and other insects.

While topical and aromatic use is generally considered safe, patchouli should not be taken internally, as there is no know safe dosage.

15. **Peppermint:** Peppermint is highly stimulating, being used to help increase energy and combat lethargy. Likewise, peppermint oil is valuable for boosting levels of creativity and concentration, as well as promoting an overall sense of mental alertness. Its energy is highly purifying, so it can be diffused throughout a room or area to remove any residual negative energy, or simply put a few drops in your bathwater after a long, stressful day to remove any excess baggage that may be following you around.

    Inhaling peppermint oil not only boosts energy levels, it can help to quell nausea and prevent motion sickness. Likewise, peppermint oil has been proven to alleviate migraine headaches while also carrying some mild respiratory benefits when applied to the chest. Peppermint oil is highly irritating to mice, spiders and ticks. Place a few cotton balls soaked in the oil in the corners of your home to guard against any unwelcome visitors or dilute the oil and use it on your clothing and backpack during hikes. It is important to note that peppermint oil is highly invigorating, thus it should not be used in any form less than five hours before you are planning on going to bed.

    Peppermint oil can be diluted with water for its analgesic and antibiotic effects as a mouthwash as well.

16. **Rose:** Just as jasmine oil is particularly beneficial for women, rose oil is the same. Not only does it help to alleviate feelings of stress, anxiety and depression, rose oil also helps to enhance beauty, attracts love and increases feelings of self-esteem. Diffusing the scent throughout a home is said to prevent against any sort of domestic arguments, while adding a few drops of the fragrance to one's bathwater is said to increase female sexuality and even promote fertility!
    Rose oil can also be used as a powerful astringent and anti-acne tool. In fact, women are encouraged to mix three or four drops of rose water in with boiling hot water and hang their heads over the steam in order to promote physical beauty and combat the external signs of aging.

17. **Rosemary:** Rosemary oils is one of the most powerful natural mental stimulants currently available on the market. A simple whiff of rosemary oil is invaluable in providing grounding and stability while promoting wisdom and increasing creativity. Students and professionals alike can benefit

from using rosemary oil to improve levels of concentration and memory retention while improving mental clarity.

Rosemary oil is showing promise in helping to preserve the memory of patients with Alzheimer's disease. It also has some pain-relieving effects when applied to tired or sore muscles.

Rosemary oil should not be used in any form by pregnant or nursing women. It should also be avoided by anyone with epilepsy or other convulsive disorders, as well as people with hypertension.

18. **Sandalwood:** Sandalwood oil carries some very strong magical connotations with it. It is believed to assist with opening an avenue to the spiritual realms, promoting wisdom, assisting in acts of divination and promoting an overall strong sense of connection to the divine. For this reason, sandalwood oil is a particularly valuable addition to all sorts of religious and spiritual ceremonies, as it helps to establish a clear connection between the individual mind and the divine. Sandalwood is also heavily associated with sexuality and passion as well. Particularly in regards to men, it restores virility and endurance while increasing levels of passion. Add a few drops of sandalwood oil to the bedsheets in order to loosen sexual inhibitions and encourage erotic play or wear the fragrance on the clothing to attract the attention of potential female suitors.

On a therapeutic level, sandalwood oil helps to relieve depressive symptoms as well as stabilizing the mood swings associated with premenstrual syndrome. Sandalwood also has sedative and calming properties, meaning that it can be used to promote a restful night's sleep as well. Sandalwood oil can also assist with alleviating muscle tension and inflammation when applied topically. It reduces the severity and discoloration of bruises, and can also combat fungal infections, such as athlete's foot.

19. Tea Tree: Tea tree oil is one of the most valuable natural substances in existence. If you decide to work with only one essential oil, tea tree is the most beneficial choice. Not only does the aroma assist with improving mental function by encouraging clarity and boosting creative energies, the medicinal benefits are virtually unparalleled.

Tea tree oil is one of the most powerful topical anti-biotics and anti-fungal agents available. Not only does the oil kill germs on contact, it is a powerful repellent for biting insects, such as mosquitos and ticks. Tea tree oil is also a remarkable topical analgesic. It can be applied to fresh stings or bug bites for a numbing effect or use it on ingrown toenails to eliminate inflammation and infection while the nail is growing out.

Quick Ailment Reference Guide

If you're ever stuck for which oil to use for which ailment, then just use this chapter as a reference.

Alleviates Anxiety: Angelica, bergamot, chamomile, frankincense, jasmine, lavender, marjoram and rose.

Analgesic: Tea Tree

Anti-fungal: Patchouli, Sandalwood and tea tree.

Anti-inflammatory: Sandalwood and tea tree.

Astringent: Rose

Attracts Love: Cinnamon, ginger, jasmine, rose and sandalwood.

Boosts Creativity: Angelica, cinnamon, peppermint and rosemary.

Clarity: Angelica, cedar, cinnamon, eucalyptus, rosemary and tea tree.

Cleanses the Liver: Bergamot

Cleanses the Kidneys: Sandalwood

Cleanses the Spleen: Bergamot

Combats Depression: Angelica, basil, bergamot, frankincense, ginger, jasmine, lavender, rose and sandalwood.

Combats Migraines: Angelica, basil, eucalyptus, lavender and peppermint.

Cures Bruises: Chamomile and Sandalwood.

Dental Aid: Frankincense and peppermint.

Digestive Aid: Ginger, marjoram and peppermint.

Enhances Divination: Sandalwood

Febrifuge: Eucalyptus

Grounding: Patchouli and rosemary.

Heals Burns: Lavender

Improves Respiratory Function: Angelica, cedar, eucalyptus, jasmine, marjoram and peppermint.

Increases Appetite: Basil and bergamot.

Increases Circulation: Cinnamon, ginger and marjoram.

Increases Concentration: Angelica, eucalyptus, lemon, rosemary and tea tree.

Increases Confidence: Cinnamon, ginger and rose.

Increases Energy: Angelica, basil, cinnamon, ginger, lemon and peppermint.

Increases Sexuality: Cinnamon, frankincense, ginger, jasmine, patchouli and sandalwood.

Laxative: Marjoram

Memory Retention: Rosemary

Menstrual Aid: Jasmine, marjoram and sandalwood.

Natural Cleaning Agent: Lemon and tea tree.

Prevents Acne: Chamomile and rose.

Prevents Nightmares: Chamomile and lavender.

Promotes Good Luck: Basil and cinnamon.

Promotes Happiness: Basil, bergamot, ginger, lavender and lemon.

Prosperity: Basil, chamomile and cinnamon.

Protection: Cedar

Purification: Cedar and peppermint.

Relieves Nausea: Basil, ginger and peppermint.

Relieves Stress: Bergamot, chamomile, frankincense, jasmine, lavender and marjoram.

Repels Insects: Chamomile, patchouli, peppermint and tea tree.

Sleep Aid: Chamomile, frankincense, jasmine, lavender and sandalwood.

Spiritual Awareness: Cedar and sandalwood.

Stability: Patchouli and rosemary.

Strengthens the Immune System: Cinnamon, frankincense, lemon and patchouli.

Wisdom: Cedar, rosemary and sandalwood.

Creating Your Own Essential Oil Blends - DIY Recipes

Once you begin to experiment with essential oils, you may become tempted to begin creating your own specialized blends. One of the most important components in creating your own blends is to be sure you are storing them properly. You will need small glass bottles that are not tinted, as exposure to direct sunlight can alter the oil's compounds. Instead, elect for bottles that are dark blue or amber tinted in color.

From here, you want to fill each bottle with approximately two tablespoons of a quality carrier oil, the two best are almond oil and jojoba oil but you can also use apricot kernel oil. This is the base that you will use to construct any of the following recipes. It is important to store these mixtures in a cool, dry area, and be sure to shake them well before using. These essential blends rely on the concept of synergy. This means that one or more essential oils are combined due to their ability to work in harmony to treat a single need. In theory, their combined power is stronger than the single oil on its own.

Some of the most practical, popular essential oil recipes are as follows:

1. **Anxiety Eliminator 1**

   3 drops jasmine

   3 drops rose

   3 drops frankincense

   Add to bathwater each night to promote restful sleep and relief from night-terrors or diffuse throughout the room for an overall sense of safety and well-being. Those who suffer from anxiety attacks may benefit from anointing their clothing with this blend or sprinkling it on their pillowcases and bedsheets.

2. **Anxiety Eliminator 2**

   2 drops bergamot

   2 drops marjoram

   3 drops lavender

This is a wonderful concoction for eliminating a generalized sense of anxiety in both children and adults. It also assists with promoting happiness and promoting focus, which makes it particularly beneficial for anointing children's school bags and school clothes.

3. **Instant Calm**

   4 drops lavender

   2 drops angelica

   2 drops marjoram

   This is an ideal blend for anyone who suffers from panic attacks. Simply take a small whiff of the blend for instant soothing, or use it in your bathwater at night to prevent against a racing mind or pointless worrying.

4. **Nature's Antidepressant**

   3 drops lavender

   2 drops sandalwood

   2 drops rose

   2 drops bergamot

   This is a wonderful oil blend for anyone who suffers from depression, obsessive tendencies or other mood disorders. It helps to promote a gentle aura of happiness when diffused throughout an area, or it can be worn on the clothing as a way of naturally uplifting the spirit.

5. **Attracting Love**

   2 drops jasmine

   2 drops patchouli

   2 drops sandalwood

   1 drop cinnamon

   Sprinkle amongst the bedsheet or diffuse throughout the bedroom to increase the libido while lowering inhibitions.

6. **Happiness Blend**

   2 drops bergamot

   2 drops lemon

   2 drops lavender

   Diffuse through a room to promote an overall sense of joy and contentment.

7. **Immunity Boost**

   2 drops lemon

   2 drops eucalyptus

   2 drops cinnamon

   Diffuse throughout the household to promote overall good health.

8. **Natural Insect Repellent**

   4 drops tea tree oil

   4 drops patchouli

   Mix with three cups of water and spray skin, clothing and bedding liberally to avoid ticks, mosquitos and other pests.

9. **Natural Mouse/Spider Repellent**

   4 drops peppermint oil

   2 drops tea tree oil

   Use the mixture to soak a cotton ball. Place one cotton ball in all of the areas of the home to discourage pests.

10. **Natural Sleep Aid**

    2 drops chamomile

    2 drops jasmine

    2 drops sandalwood

    Diffuse the mixture throughout a room or sprinkle it onto bedsheets to ensure a good night's sleep.

11. **Nature's Housekeeper**

4 drops lemon oil

4 drops tea tree

Place the blend in about two cups of water and mix in a spray bottle for an excellent, all-natural cleaning remedy that is non-toxic and safe for children and pets. Spray on kitchen counters, in the bathtub, toilet, sink or any other area to clean while preventing bacteria and germs.

12. Sweet Dreams

4 drops lavender

4 drops chamomile

2 drops jasmine

A simple whiff of this blend before bedtime helps to promote restlessness or diffuse it through the bedroom an hour before bedtime to ensure that children receive a deep, pleasant sleep.

13. Nature's Excedrin

4 drops lavender

2 drops peppermint

2 drops eucalyptus

The best way to use this formula is to simply inhale it at the first sign of a migraine onset. Even if you are not able to use it in the beginning phases, taking a small whiff every ten minutes or so will help to alleviate the worst of the symptoms. Those who are especially prone to stress migraines can combine two drops of lavender to the solution to help promote calmness as well.

14. Nausea Relief

3 drops ginger

3 drops peppermint

Inhale the scent directly from the bottle to alleviate the symptoms of motion sickness, or simply diffuse the mixture through a room to alleviate upset stomachs associated with morning sickness, hangover or digestive issues.

15. Passion Booster

3 drops cinnamon

2 drops rose

2 drops sandalwood

An ideal date-night blend, this is a wonderful addition to a couple's bath or massage, as it arouses the libido and promotes an aura of romance and sexuality. Sprinkle the mixture onto your bedsheet or clothes for the same effect or diffuse the scent throughout a room and watch the sparks fly!

16. Prosperity/Money Drawing Blend

3 drops chamomile

3 drops cinnamon

Use as a hand wash to increase monetary flow or use the oil blend to anoint the purse or wallet for the same purpose. The mixture can also be sprinkled around the house to promote overall good luck.

17. Protection

4 drops cedar oil

Use this mixture to anoint clothing to ward against accidents and other danger, particularly when traveling. This same mixture can be used on objects to prevent them from becoming damaged or stolen. When diffused in an area or sprinkled around the perimeter of a room, it guards against negative energies and wards off any malevolent entities that may be lurking nearby.

18. Bruise Remover

3 drops chamomile

3 drops sandalwood

Mix the oil blend with a cup of cold water and soak a rag in it to create a kind of compress. Drape the cloth over the bruised area for a few minutes to help improve discoloration and to discourage inflammation. Chamomile oil can be very irritating to the skin, so do not attempt this remedy unless you have used it topically before with no adverse effects.

19. Respiratory Aid

2 drops eucalyptus

2 drops peppermint

Mix with a quality carrier oil and rub on the chest for a decongestant effect or diffuse throughout the room or add to bathwater to aid with mild respiratory issues.

20. The Scholar's Blend

3 drops eucalyptus

3 drops lemon

2 drops rosemary

This is an excellent scent to diffuse throughout an area in order to enhance concentration and help with memory retention. Use it while studying or reading, then carry the bottle with you and take a deep breath of it before a test or exam to boost focus and increase the ability to recall what you have learned.

21. Stress Relief

2 drops jasmine

2 drops lavender

2 drops frankincense

Diffuse throughout a room or add to bathwater to promote an environment of peacefulness, calm and tranquility.

22. Woman's Best Friend

4 drops sandalwood

4 drops jasmine

Diffuse throughout a room or wear as a scent during one's menstrual period for obtaining relief from mood swings as well as to combat cramping and fatigue. This is also an excellent mixture to sprinkle upon the bedsheets to encourage fertility and increase female libido.

Conclusion

And there we go, I hope you've enjoyed this book and that it's proved valuable to you. I urge you to try out some of the recipes listed as well.

One important thing to remember is to only buy high quality essential oils, sometimes cheaper brands pass off "massage oils" as being essential oils - but this is not the case. A surefire way to tell if an oil is fake is if they feel greasy or thick. The exception to this rule is sandalwood, which naturally has a thicker consistency.

Whatever your reason for using essential oils, they are a fantastic, natural way to remedy various ailments, both physical and mental.

Essential oils are quickly gaining recognition for their tremendous healing properties. There is absolutely no question that essential oils help treat the symptoms of different diseases as effectively or more than the drugs which are administered by pharmaceutical companies.
So best of luck to you in your essential oil journey - and I wish you all the best.

One final note, if this book has been useful to you - I'd really appreciate it if you left it a review on Amazon.

Thanks,
Lauren

www.ingramcontent.com/pod-product-compliance
Lightning Source LLC
Chambersburg PA
CBHW080629030426

42336CB00018B/3129